Table of contents

Introduction

My name is Michael and I'm currently a male model with over 10,000 subscribers on YouTube. I've made over 2,000 from modelling and over 1,000 from YouTube. I've generated thousands of pounds from my looks and I want to teach you how to do the same.

My journey began when I realised that I had an unfair advantage, my looks. I was in a bad place in life when I realised this, a homeless hostel surrounded by crackheads. I had barely any money to my name and a bad relationship with my family. I also had just been released from prison for armed robbery.

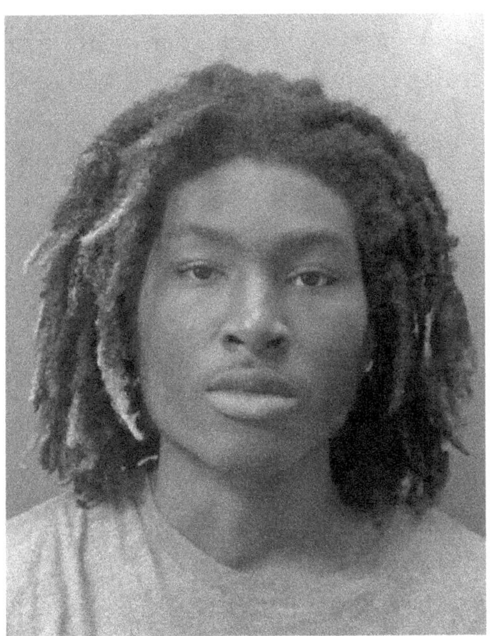

My childhood was quite bad. I had a negligent father who wasn't around and my mother is one of the worst people I know in life. My mother would constantly leave me homeless in the streets or with family members. I have been in both foster care and residential care due to my mother. I was never a bad kid; my mother never really wanted me if I'm being honest. My mother would leave me home alone with my younger sibling while she went out to party, all the time.

My mother had a sister who also lived with me and my mother alongside her kid. My aunty also would call police on me and have me kicked out for stuff like telling her kid to go to bed at 23:00 pm (He was 11 btw).

I wasn't really focused in school due to my chaotic household. This left me finishing school wondering where my life would end up. I went to a basketball college after high school but didn't find much success due to my disability. I have a disability that causes me severe pain when I'm on my feet for long periods of time. I still chased my dreams of becoming a basketball player until I realised I couldn't no more.

I decided to get a job after taking a year off college trying to figure out what I was going to do with my life. After a couple months on the job, I committed an armed robbery which resulted in me having to serve a 2-year sentence. I had quite bad mental health at the time and I was also very angry at my childhood. After I finished my 2-year sentence I was in a homeless hostel around the worst of the worst people. Someone literally tried to rob my bike, karma huh? Before I was in the homeless hostel, I was in a temporary accommodation for a couple months.

I began working out to keep a positive mindset while I was in the hostel. I came across a book named "Predictable Irrationality" which taught me about blind consistency and how I was just doing things just to do them. Reading this book helped me break from my old habits and start going to the gym. To sum up blind consistency it refers to the rigid and unthinking adherence to a pattern, rule, or routine without considering whether it is still appropriate or effective. This was thought pattern I had when I wasn't doing well in life. Blind consistency can be applied in various contexts, such as in decision-making, habits, or organizational practices.

When someone follows a course of action out of "blind consistency," they do so without questioning its relevance, even if circumstances have changed or the approach is no longer beneficial. This behaviour can lead to inefficiency, missed opportunities, or negative outcomes (which I kept experiencing) because it prioritizes sticking to a previous commitment or habit over adapting to new information or conditions.

When I began changing my thought patterns, I started seeing changes that made me feel more positive about my current situation. If you know anyone that has been in a homeless hostel it's quite depressing. For those who don't quite know what a homeless hostel is like… people often sleep in dormitory-style rooms with multiple beds, which means little to no privacy. Personal belongings are typically stored in shared areas or lockers, leading to a lack of personal space. Most people there are recovering drug addicts or in pretty negative places in their life. Scroll to the next page to see the state of my accommodation that eventually caused me to move to a homeless hostel…

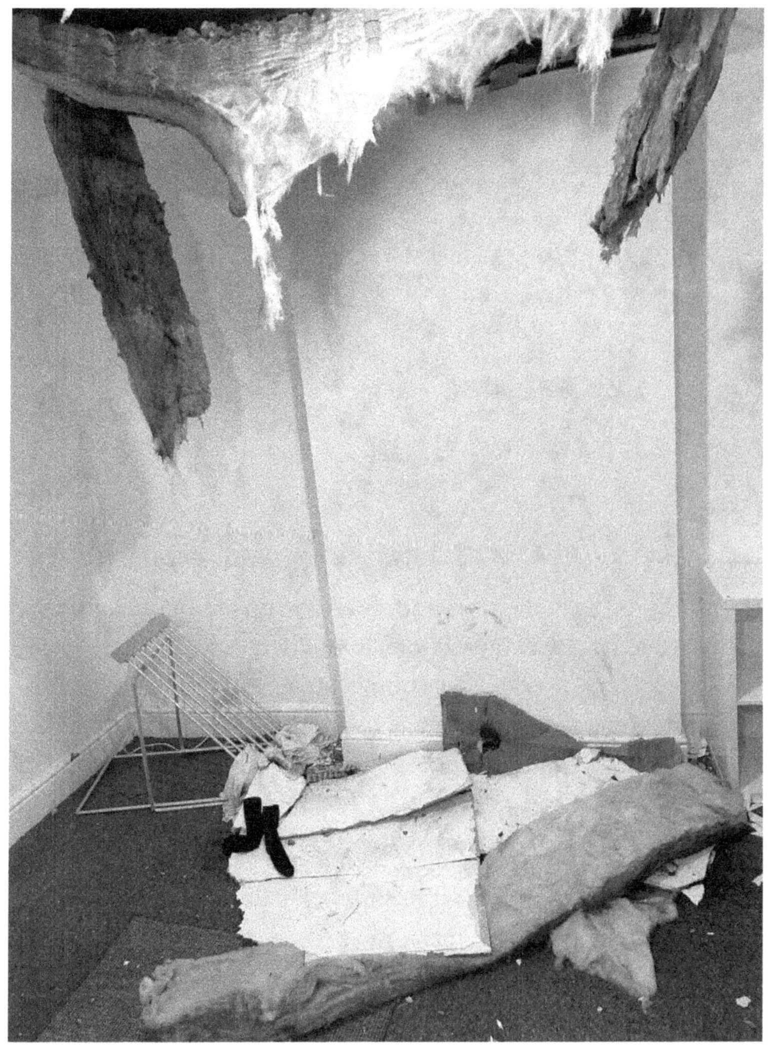

I was going through it living in the homeless hostel so I decided to look for something positive to do so I started making reactions on my YouTube channel Suave Shawty. I was also dealing with multiple women and encountering similar experiences with these women. This is when I decided to make my first handsome men's game video. The video was about maximising your looks even if you're already attractive. I was making fashion videos before this but they didn't really take off.

As soon as I made that video, I saw a couple hundred views which wasn't new to me at that point. It was when I made my "Handsome men should avoid these types of women at all cost" video, that I saw my first 1,000 views. I woke up the following day after posting and was filled with excitement. This was when I realised there's an audience for giving game about women to attractive men.

I've been grinding ever since and now I'm at 11,200 subscribers and have generated thousands.

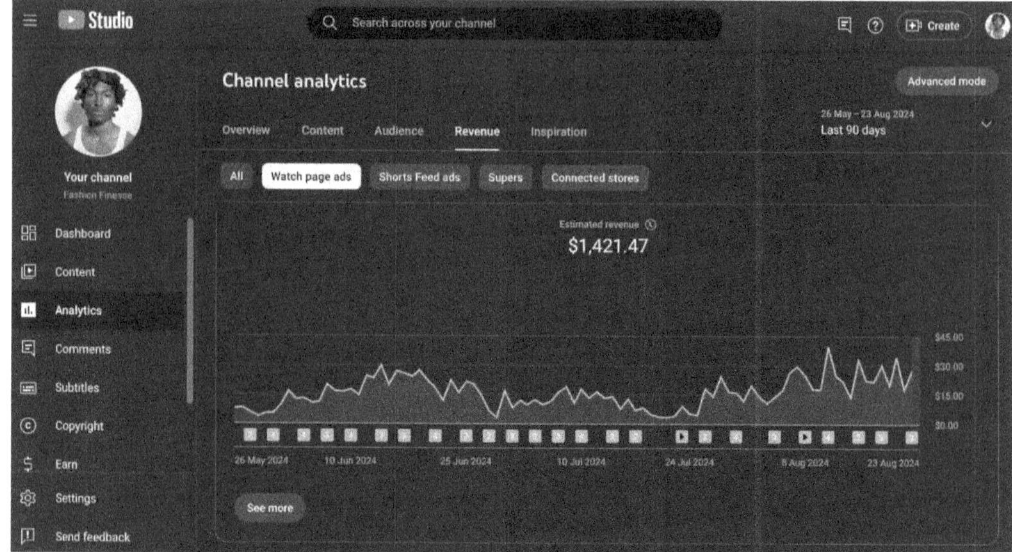

I was heavily self-improving at the time and when you do this, your confidence goes up. Due to this I decided to do a walk-in at a local modelling agency. I got rejected at the first agency I went to; I could tell this was coming because they barely looked me in the eye. I decided to brush my shoulders and go to another agency 10 minutes away. I got signed on the spot! I then began incorporating my modelling with my channel, that's when my YouTube really started growing.

I believe this is due to my "unfair advantage". I'm a male model talking about the experience of attractive men, I'm a trusted source unlike guys who are just saying they're attractive. With this book, I want show you how to get more out of life with your unfair advantage.

Unfair Advantage

As I explained in the introduction my unfair advantage is that I'm a male model talking about the experience of attractive men. An average looking guy is going to have as much authority as me when talking about attraction. For you to realise what your personal unfair advantage is, we have to first understand what exactly an unfair advantage means.

An unfair advantage refers to a condition, resource, or opportunity that gives one person or group a significant benefit over others in a way that is not justifiable or ethical. It typically implies that the advantage was not earned through merit, hard work, or legitimate means, and it may involve exploiting loopholes, insider knowledge, or favourable circumstances that others do not have access to. Unfair advantages can create imbalances in competition, opportunities, or outcomes, leading to an unequal playing field where some parties are at a distinct disadvantage.

Examples include:

- **Insider Information**: Using non-public knowledge in the stock market to gain financial benefits.
- **Nepotism**: Gaining job opportunities or promotions due to family connections rather than qualifications.
- **Regulatory Loopholes**: Exploiting legal gaps that others are unaware of to gain financial or competitive benefits.
- **Exclusive Access**: Having access to resources, technology, or networks that others cannot reach.

I want you to ask yourself, what's my unfair advantage? For example, you could be a guy who wants to be a fitness influencer. Your unfair advantage is that people will trust your fitness advice if you're in shape and attractive, more so than a "science bro" who knows everything about working out but he isn't attractive. The guys making the most money in the fitness industry aren't the guys with the most fitness knowledge. I'm going to let you think about that for a second.

Businesses use attractive people as an unfair advantage all the time. When Gucci does a campaign, this is exactly what they're doing. Their using attractive models to sell their product. If the owner of Gucci modelled the clothes, do you think they would sell? Now it may not be that extreme nowadays since everyone can get attractive models but, you better believe that having an attractive model was a serious unfair advantage when fashion was just beginning to rise.

Fashion brands still use an unfair advantage in other ways. For example, if you have a popular model wearing your clothes on a runway this is an unfair advantage. Popular models have more freedom when it comes to selecting jobs. Someone like Alton Mason (male model) can pick what brand he wants to work for. This would give the brand he chooses to work for an unfair advantage over the competition, when selling their clothes. Still haven't thought of your unfair advantage yet? Don't worry, it took me awhile. When you do find your unfair advantage, it's like winning the lottery.

Why Using Attraction for Success Is Your Unfair Advantage

People treat human beings according to their attraction. Sounds crazy right? What if I told you that as shallow as it seems, this is actually true. Statistics show that attractive people are more favourable especially when it comes to jobs and dating. Astrid Hopfensitz, Professor in organizational behaviour, EM Lyon Business School. She says "In today's fiercely competitive job market, the economic advantages of beauty are undeniable. Numerous studies have shown that attractive individuals benefit from a beauty bonus and earn higher salaries on average.

Psychology Today states "Attractiveness is positively related to employment opportunity, wages, and performance evaluations. A penalty based on same-sex bias occurs when pretty people are judged more harshly by those of similar gender".

Forbes states "Attractive people have an advantage in the job search and advancing in their careers. We talk about all types of biases, but largely ignore the fact that decisions are made based upon how someone looks. While deep down, we all kind of know that this is sort of true, a new University of Buffalo study confirms this inconvenient and uncomfortable fact.

Separately, a Harvard Study previously confirmed, "Workers of above average beauty earn about 10 to 15% more than workers of below-average beauty. The size of this beauty premium is economically significant and comparable to the race and gender gaps in the U.S. labour market." For example, you tend to see generally tall men as CEOs of major corporations and winning presidential candidates.

The findings of the UB study show, "Attractive people are more likely to get hired, receive better evaluations and get paid more." The results indicate that there is something called a "beauty premium" that exists across professions.

Min-Hsuan Tu, assistant professor in the organization and human resources department and lead author on the study, said, "People like pretty or handsome people—that's traditionally viewed as a bias, because pretty or handsome people could get more opportunities, we give them more resources, so they're more likely to be successful."

As we can see with these studies, attractive people are definitely favoured when it comes to opportunity in life. So, the question is now are you going to take the opportunity/unfair advantage or leave it?

My Weekly Guide to Maintain Peak Attraction

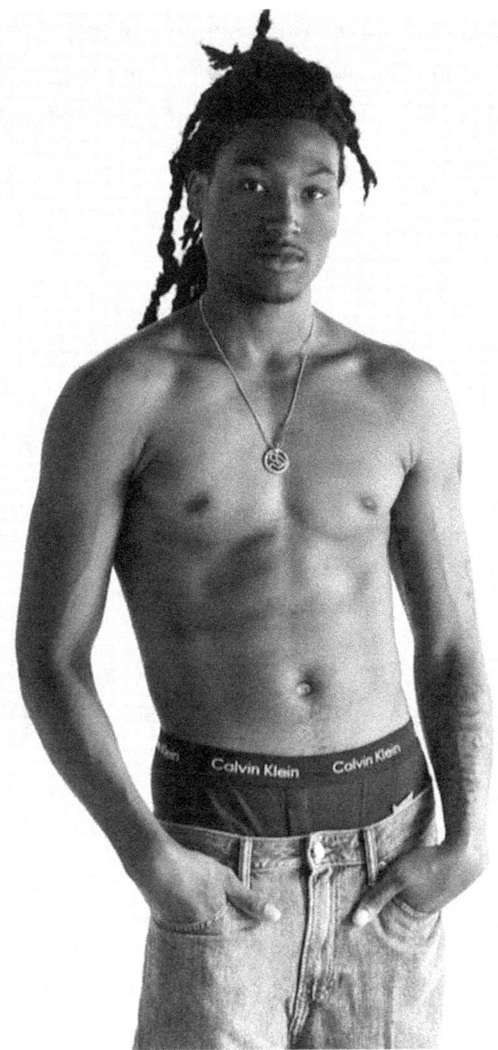

I have a weekly routine that helps me maintain peak attraction. This routine contains fitness, skincare, health and wellness.

Weekly Fitness Routine

- **Monday**: Arms (3x8 Bicep curls, 3x8 Seated Bicep Curls, 3x8 Close Grip Pullups, 3x8 Shoulder press and 3x8 Overhead triceps extension into 3x8 Bicep curls)
- **Tuesday**: Chest (3x8 Flat, Upper and Lower dumbbell press. 3x8 Chest Fly, 3x8 Hanging Leg Raise and 3x8 sit ups with the lower bench, holding 5KG to my core)
- **Wednesday**: Legs and Back (3x8 Lunges, 3x8 Leg curl, 3x8 Prone Leg Curl, 3x8 Wide Grip Pullups and 3x8 Lat Pull Down)

- **Thursday**: Arms (3x8 Bicep curls, 3x8 Seated Bicep Curls, 3x8 Close Grip Pullups, 3x8 shoulder raises into 3x8 Bicep curls and 3x8 Shoulder press)
- **Friday**: Chest (3x8 Flat, Upper and Lower bench. 3x8 Push ups into Dips. 3x8 Hanging Leg Raise and 3x8 Russian Twists.)

Daily Skincare Routine

Morning:

1. **Cleanser**
   - Use a gentle cleanser suited to your skin type to remove overnight oils and impurities.
   - **Example**: Gel cleanser for oily skin, cream cleanser for dry skin.
2. **Serum**
   - Choose a serum that targets specific concerns like hydration, brightening, or anti-aging.
   - **Example**: Vitamin C serum for brightening, hyaluronic acid for hydration.
3. **Moisturizer**
   - Locks in moisture and keeps your skin hydrated.
   - **Example**: Lightweight moisturizer for oily skin, rich cream for dry skin.

Evening:

4. **Cleanser**
   - Use the same cleanser as in the morning to clean your face.
5. **Exfoliant** (2-3 times a week)
   - Helps remove dead skin cells and unclogs pores.
6. **Treatment/Serum**
   - Apply any specific treatments for acne, hyperpigmentation, or anti-aging.
7. **Eye Cream** (Optional)
   - Helps to address concerns like puffiness, dark circles, or fine lines around the eyes.
8. **Moisturizer or Night Cream**
   - Use a slightly heavier moisturizer or night cream to repair your skin overnight.
9. **Face Mask** (1-2 times a week)
   - Use a mask that addresses your specific concerns.
10. **Exfoliation** (as mentioned above)
    - Stick to exfoliating 2-3 times per week to avoid over-exfoliation.
11. **Deep Hydration** (Optional)

- o   Use an overnight hydrating mask or a hydrating serum for extra moisture.

Additional Tips:

- **Patch Test**: Always patch test new products to avoid irritation.
- **Consistency**: Stick to your routine for at least a few weeks to see results.
- **Diet & Hydration**: Maintain a balanced diet and drink plenty of water.
- **Adjust for Seasons**: Your routine may need adjustments for different seasons.

Weekly Food Routine

- **Breakfast**: 7 eggs and a banana.
- **Snack**: 3x Driod Mango.
- **Lunch**: 1,000 calorie fruit mix (peanuts, almonds and cashews) smoothie with a tea cup of oats and two scoops of peanut butter.
- **Snack**: banana.
- **Dinner**: 3x Roast chicken and medium sized portion of rice with a banana.

Morning Schedule

5:00 AM - Wake Up

- **Avoid Snoozing**: Get out of bed as soon as your alarm goes off to start your day on a proactive note.
- **Hydrate**: Drink a glass of water to kickstart your metabolism and rehydrate after a night's sleep.

5:10 AM - Stretch or Light Exercise

- **Stretching**: Spend 5-10 minutes stretching to wake up your muscles and improve circulation.
- **Exercise (Optional)**: If you prefer working out in the morning, do 20-30 minutes of moderate exercise like jogging, yoga, or bodyweight exercises.

5:30 AM - Personal Hygiene

- **Shower and Grooming**: A warm shower can help you feel refreshed. Follow up with brushing your teeth, skincare, and grooming.

5:45 AM - Breakfast

- **Healthy Breakfast**: Eat a balanced breakfast that includes protein, healthy fats, and complex carbohydrates. For example, eggs with whole-grain toast and avocado, or oatmeal with fruit and nuts.

6:15 AM - Plan Your Day

- **Review Your To-Do List**: Take a few minutes to look over your tasks and set priorities.
- **Mindfulness (Optional)**: Practice 5-10 minutes of meditation, deep breathing, or journaling to focus your mind.

6:30 AM - Start Your Day

- **Work or Study**: Begin your day's primary activities, such as work, study, or other responsibilities, feeling energized and focused.

Sleep Schedule

9:00 PM - Personal Hygiene

- **Nighttime Routine**: Brush your teeth, wash your face, and follow your evening skincare routine.

9:20 PM - Wind Down

- **Dim the Lights**: Start lowering the lights to signal to your body that it's time to relax.
- **Screen Time**: Avoid screens (phones, computers, TVs) to reduce exposure to blue light, which can interfere with melatonin production.

9:40 PM - Relaxing Activity

- **Reading or Journaling**: Engage in a relaxing activity like reading a book, journaling, or listening to calming music.
- **Light Stretching or Yoga**: Gentle stretching can help relieve muscle tension and prepare your body for sleep.

10:00 PM - Bedtime

- **Get Into Bed**: Aim to be in bed with lights out by 10:00 PM.
- **Sleep Environment**: Ensure your room is cool, quiet, and dark. Consider using a sleep mask or white noise machine if needed.

10:00 PM - 5:00 AM - Sleep

- **Aim for 7-9 Hours**: Quality sleep is crucial for recovery and overall health. Try to maintain this schedule consistently, even on weekends.

Additional Tips:

- **Consistency**: Stick to your schedule as much as possible, even on weekends, to regulate your body's internal clock.
- **Caffeine**: Avoid caffeine in the afternoon and evening to prevent it from interfering with your sleep.

I have been following this routine for the past year. This routine has contributed not only to my attractiveness but, my success in life.

Guide To Becoming a Model

Becoming a male model involves a combination of physical preparation, professional development, networking, and industry knowledge. Here's a step-by-step guide to help you get started:

1. Understand the Industry

- **Research**: Familiarize yourself with the different types of male modelling, including fashion (runway, editorial), commercial (advertising, print), fitness, and body part modelling (e.g., hands).
- **Study Successful Models**: Look at the careers of successful male models to understand what worked for them. Follow their social media, read interviews, and observe their portfolios.

2. Physical Preparation

- **Fitness and Grooming**: Maintain a healthy, toned physique appropriate for the type of modelling you're pursuing. Regular exercise, a balanced diet, and skincare are essential.

- **Height and Measurements**: While there are opportunities for different body types, high fashion typically requires a height of 5'11" to 6'2" with a lean build. Commercial modelling offers more flexibility.
- **Skincare**: Clear skin is important. Establish a daily skincare routine, stay hydrated, and address any skin issues with a dermatologist if needed.
- **Grooming**: Keep hair neat, maintain facial hair as required (or clean-shaven if preferred), and consider teeth whitening if necessary.

3. Build a Portfolio

- **Professional Photos**: Invest in professional headshots and full-body shots. A diverse portfolio should show various looks, including casual, formal, and fitness shots.
- **Test Shoots**: Collaborate with photographers for test shoots. These are unpaid shoots that help you build your portfolio and gain experience.

4. Gain Experience

- **Local Opportunities**: Start with local modelling gigs, such as fashion shows, photoshoots, or promotional events, to gain experience.
- **Networking**: Attend industry events, fashion shows, and modelling workshops to meet professionals and other models.

5. Find Representation

- **Research Agencies**: Look for reputable modelling agencies that represent male models. Check their requirements for submissions, which usually include photos, measurements, and a brief bio.
- **Submit Applications**: Submit your portfolio to multiple agencies. If possible, attend open casting calls where agencies look for new talent.
- **Avoid Scams**: Be cautious of agencies or individuals who ask for large upfront fees. Legitimate agencies make money by booking jobs for you, not through fees.

6. Social Media Presence

- **Instagram and TikTok**: Use social media platforms to showcase your portfolio, lifestyle, and personality. Engage with followers and industry professionals.
- **Content Creation**: Post regularly, including behind-the-scenes shots, daily routines, and professional work. Tag brands and photographers to increase visibility.

7. Attend Castings and Auditions

- **Persistence**: Attend as many castings and auditions as possible. Rejection is common, so resilience is key.
- **Preparedness**: Always bring your portfolio, be punctual, and maintain a professional demeanour.

8. Develop Your Skills

- **Runway Training**: If you're interested in runway modelling, practice walking with confidence. Consider taking a runway class or workshop.
- **Posing Practice**: Learn how to pose for different types of shoots. Practice in front of a mirror or with a photographer.
- **Acting and Expression**: Many modelling gigs require a range of expressions. Consider taking acting classes to improve your versatility.

9. Stay Professional

- **Contracts and Payments**: Understand contracts before signing and keep track of your payments. Seek legal advice if needed.
- **Professionalism**: Be reliable, communicate clearly, and maintain a good reputation in the industry. Building strong relationships can lead to repeat bookings.

10. Continuous Improvement

- **Feedback**: Listen to feedback from photographers, agencies, and clients to improve your craft.
- **Adaptability**: The industry evolves, so stay updated on trends, maintain your physical appearance, and continue building your portfolio.

11. Consider Specialization

- **Fashion**: Focus on high fashion, runway, or editorial work if you meet the height and body type requirements.
- **Commercial**: Explore opportunities in commercial modelling, which includes advertisements and print campaigns.
- **Fitness**: If you have a well-defined physique, fitness modelling might be a good fit. This often involves working with sports brands and fitness publications.

12. Keep a Balanced Perspective

- **Mental Health**: The modelling industry can be demanding, with pressures related to appearance and competition. Prioritize your mental health, seek support when needed, and remember that rejection is part of the process.
- **Longevity**: Consider how you can sustain a long-term career. Some models transition into acting, photography, or other fashion industry roles as they age.

Conclusion

Becoming a successful male model requires dedication, persistence, and a proactive approach to personal development and networking. By following these steps and staying true to your goals, you can build a rewarding career in the modelling industry.

I want to show you what is possible if you follow all of these steps so here's some of my payments from modelling so far...

Boss Agencies Ltd
T/A Boss Model Management
33 Turner Street
Manchester
M4 1DW

VAT Reg No GB 732339247

MICAW1B   VAT Reg   GB

Michael Awoyemi

Great Britain

BOSS

All amounts shown in   Pound Sterling

26/02/2024

Payment will be in your account
on Tuesday 27th Feb 2024

Date	Inv No.	Client	Job Details	Expenses	Net Fee	VAT	Payable
06/02/2024	32016/06	BEYOND 90	Puma Fashion Show	0.00	438.00	0.00	438.00
			Job Details				
			Fittings/Rehersal				
			Show				
			Overtime				

Total remittance: **£438.00**

Boss Agencies Ltd
T/A Boss Model Management
33 Turner Street
Manchester
M4 1DW

VAT Reg No   GB   732339247

MICAW1B   VAT Reg   GB

Michael Awoyemi

Great Britain

BOSS

All amounts shown in   Pound Sterling

03/11/2023

Payment will be in your account
on Monday 6th Nov 2023

Please keep this remittance safe, as you may need it for tax purposes

Date	Inv No.	Client	Job Details	Expenses	Net Fee	VAT	Payable
26/09/2023	30777	JD SPORTS FASHION PLC	Ecomme Shoot	0.00	487.50	0.00	487.50
			Job Details				
			Full Day				

Total remittance: £487.50

Boss Agencies Ltd
T/A Boss Model Management
33 Turner Street
Manchester
M4 1DW

VAT Reg No   GB   732339247

MICAW1B   VAT Reg   GB

Michael Awoyemi

Great Britain

BOSS

All amounts shown in   Pound Sterling

30/05/2024

Payment will be in your account
on Friday 31st May 2024

Date	Inv No.	Client	Job Details	Expenses	Net Fee	VAT	Payable
27/03/2024	32527/01	DE MONTFORT UNIVERSITY	Photoshoot	104.00	112.50	0.00	216.50
			Job Details				
			10.00 - 17.00				
		Exps Train		104.00			

Total remittance: £216.50

Alternative ways to get paid for your looks

If you're a man looking to monetize your appearance outside of traditional modelling, there are several alternative ways to get paid using your looks. Here's a guide to some of the most viable options:

1. Social Media Influencer

- **Platforms**: Instagram, TikTok, YouTube, etc.
- **How It Works**: Build a following around your personal style, fitness journey, grooming tips, or lifestyle. Once you have an audience, brands may pay you to promote their products through sponsored posts, collaborations, or affiliate marketing.
- **Monetization**: Sponsored content, affiliate marketing, brand ambassadorships, and ad revenue.

2. Content Creation (Only Fans, Patreon, etc.)

- **Platforms**: Only Fans, Patreon, Fan house, etc.
- **How It Works**: Create exclusive content tailored to your audience. This could include fitness tips, grooming advice, or more adult-oriented content. Subscribers pay for access, and you set the pricing.
- **Monetization**: Subscription fees, tips, and paid exclusive content.

3. Fitness Coaching or Personal Training

- **How It Works**: Use your physique to promote fitness coaching services. You can offer in-person training sessions, online coaching, or create workout programs. A fit appearance helps attract clients and build credibility.
- **Monetization**: Client sessions, online fitness programs, eBooks, and merchandise.

4. Brand Ambassador

- **How It Works**: Partner with brands that align with your look and lifestyle, such as grooming products, clothing, or fitness gear. Promote these products online or at events.
- **Monetization**: Paid partnerships, free products, and commissions from sales.

5. Acting and Extra Work

- **How It Works**: Use your appearance to secure roles in commercials, TV shows, movies, or music videos. Even if you're not the lead, you can earn money as an extra or in minor roles.
- **Monetization**: Acting gigs, extra work fees, and residuals from commercial work.

6. Fashion Blogging or Vlogging

- **Platforms**: YouTube, Instagram, TikTok, personal blogs.
- **How It Works**: Share your fashion insights, style tips, and grooming routines. Build an audience interested in men's fashion, and monetize through ads, sponsored content, and partnerships.
- **Monetization**: Ad revenue, sponsored posts, affiliate marketing, and product collaborations.

7. Hair and Grooming Model

- **How It Works**: Model for barbershops, hairstylists, or grooming brands. This could involve photoshoots, tutorials, or promotional events. Your hairstyle or beard could become a brand's signature look.
- **Monetization**: Paid modelling gigs, free services, and product endorsements.

8. Live Streaming (Gaming, Lifestyle, etc.)

- **Platforms**: Twitch, YouTube Live, Facebook Gaming.
- **How It Works**: Stream content such as gaming, fitness routines, or lifestyle tips. An attractive appearance can help you stand out and build a following.
- **Monetization**: Donations, subscriptions, sponsorships, and ad revenue.

9. Model for Art Classes or Workshops

- **How It Works**: Pose for art classes where students practice drawing or painting the human form. This is often part-time and can be a unique way to monetize your appearance.
- **Monetization**: Hourly fees for modelling sessions.

10. Fitness and Physique Competitions

- **How It Works**: Participate in bodybuilding, physique, or fitness competitions. Winning or placing well can lead to cash prizes, sponsorship deals, and exposure in fitness magazines or brands.
- **Monetization**: Competition prizes, sponsorships, and endorsement deals.

11. Event Hosting or Promoting

- **How It Works**: Leverage your looks and charisma to host or promote events, such as nightclub parties, brand launches, or charity events. Being the face of an event can attract attendees and generate income.
- **Monetization**: Appearance fees, commissions, or sponsorships.

12. Grooming and Style Consultant

- **How It Works**: Use your knowledge of men's grooming and fashion to offer consulting services. Help clients improve their style, grooming routines, or overall appearance.
- **Monetization**: Consulting fees, product commissions, and personalized styling packages.

13. Modelling for Stock Photos

- **How It Works**: Pose for stock photo agencies that need a variety of images featuring everyday scenarios. These photos are used in advertisements, websites, and publications.
- **Monetization**: Payment per session and potential royalties from photo usage.

14. Virtual Fitness or Grooming Workshops

- **How It Works**: Conduct online workshops teaching fitness routines, grooming techniques, or fashion advice. Use platforms like Zoom or Instagram Live to reach a broad audience.
- **Monetization**: Workshop fees, donations, and ongoing subscriptions.

15. Companion Services

- **How It Works**: Offer your services as a companion for social events, dinners, or travel, where clients pay for your company and presence. This is often about making clients feel at ease and enhancing their social experiences.

- **Monetization**: Hourly or event-based fees.

16. Digital Fashion Shows or Lookbooks

- **How It Works**: Collaborate with emerging fashion brands or designers to showcase their clothes in digital formats, such as virtual fashion shows or lookbooks. Your appearance can help brands reach wider audiences.
- **Monetization**: Paid collaborations, free clothing, and exposure.

These avenues provide diverse opportunities to monetize your looks as a man, whether through digital content, personal services, or industry-specific roles. Choose the path that best aligns with your skills, interests, and goals.

How to Get More Out of Your Life with Your Looks

Leveraging your looks as a man can open up various opportunities beyond just traditional modelling. Here's how you can get more out of life by maximizing your appearance:

1. Develop Confidence and Charisma

- **Self-Assurance**: Confidence is key to making the most of your looks. Work on self-esteem by setting and achieving personal goals, practicing self-care, and surrounding yourself with supportive people.
- **Charisma**: Cultivate charisma by improving your communication skills, maintaining a positive attitude, and showing genuine interest in others. Charisma, combined with good looks, can make you more appealing in social and professional settings.

2. Networking and Social Opportunities

- **Attend Social Events**: Use your appearance to your advantage at social gatherings, networking events, and parties. People often remember those who stand out visually, which can help you make valuable connections.
- **Cultivate a Strong Social Media Presence**: Build a polished online presence on platforms like Instagram, LinkedIn, or TikTok. A strong visual brand can attract opportunities for collaborations, partnerships, or even job offers.

3. Explore the Dating and Relationship Scene

- **Dating Apps**: Use dating apps to connect with others. A good profile picture and a well-curated bio can increase your chances of meeting interesting people.
- **First Impressions**: Your looks can make a strong first impression, but pairing them with intelligence, kindness, and a sense of humour can help you build meaningful relationships.

4. Career Advancement

- **Personal Branding**: In professional environments, appearance often plays a role in how others perceive you. Dress well, groom yourself, and maintain a confident posture to enhance your professional image.
- **Public Speaking and Leadership Roles**: Consider roles that put you in the public eye, such as public speaking, sales, or leadership. Your looks, combined with confidence and eloquence, can make you a more persuasive and memorable figure.

5. Engage in Fitness and Wellness

- **Health as a Priority**: Prioritize fitness and wellness to maintain and enhance your appearance. A healthy lifestyle not only improves your looks but also boosts energy, mood, and overall well-being.
- **Fitness Modelling or Coaching**: Consider leveraging your physique for fitness-related opportunities, such as modelling, coaching, or social media content focused on health and fitness.

6. Travel and Experiences

- **Travel Influencer**: If you love to travel, combine your looks with your experiences to become a travel influencer. Share your adventures on social media to inspire others and attract partnerships with travel brands or tourism boards.
- **Free or Discounted Opportunities**: Attractive individuals often receive perks or discounts in certain environments, such as clubs, events, or travel experiences. Use these opportunities to explore new places and experiences.

7. Media and Entertainment

- **Acting and Entertainment**: Explore opportunities in acting, hosting, or entertainment, where your looks can be a significant asset. Even if you start small, these roles can lead to larger opportunities.
- **Content Creation**: Use platforms like YouTube or TikTok to create engaging content that highlights your personality and looks. This could range from fashion and grooming tips to lifestyle vlogs.

8. Personal Development

- **Continuous Learning**: While looks can open doors, it's important to develop your skills, knowledge, and personal interests. Engage in continuous learning, whether through formal education, self-study, or life experiences, to ensure you're well-rounded and can sustain the opportunities your appearance brings.
- **Hobbies and Interests**: Cultivate hobbies that complement your looks, such as fashion design, photography, or fitness. These activities can lead to new skills, social circles, and personal fulfilment.

9. Entrepreneurial Ventures

- **Fashion and Grooming**: If you have a passion for fashion or grooming, consider starting your own brand, whether it's a clothing line, a grooming product, or a style consultancy. Your looks can help market the brand effectively.
- **Influencer Marketing**: Collaborate with brands to create content that aligns with your personal brand. As an influencer, you can leverage your looks to partner with companies, creating a lucrative side business.

10. Give Back and Inspire Others

- **Mentorship and Guidance**: Use your influence to mentor others, particularly younger individuals or those looking to enter fields like fitness, modelling, or social media. Your experiences can inspire and guide them.
- **Philanthropy**: Participate in charitable activities or causes. Your looks and public presence can help bring attention to important issues, making a positive impact on society.

11. Maximize Opportunities with Emotional Intelligence

- **Understanding Perception**: Use emotional intelligence to understand how others perceive you based on your looks and how you can navigate different social dynamics effectively.
- **Building Authentic Relationships**: Cultivate genuine relationships based on trust and mutual respect, rather than relying solely on appearance.

12. Long-Term Planning

- **Plan for the Future**: While looks can be an asset, they are just one part of your life. Think about long-term goals that go beyond appearance, such as career ambitions, financial stability, and personal happiness.
- **Diversify Your Skillset**: As you age, having a diverse skillset will help you continue to thrive in different areas of life, even as your looks change.

By combining your looks with confidence, social skills, and a focus on personal growth, you can open up a wide range of opportunities in both your personal and professional life. The content in this book has helped me turn my life from negative to positive. I've built multiple business off my looks and this book can help you do the same. I love you guys' that continually support my every move! Send me any updates on your journey to my Instagram @Mikedawiz28.

Fashion Finesse...

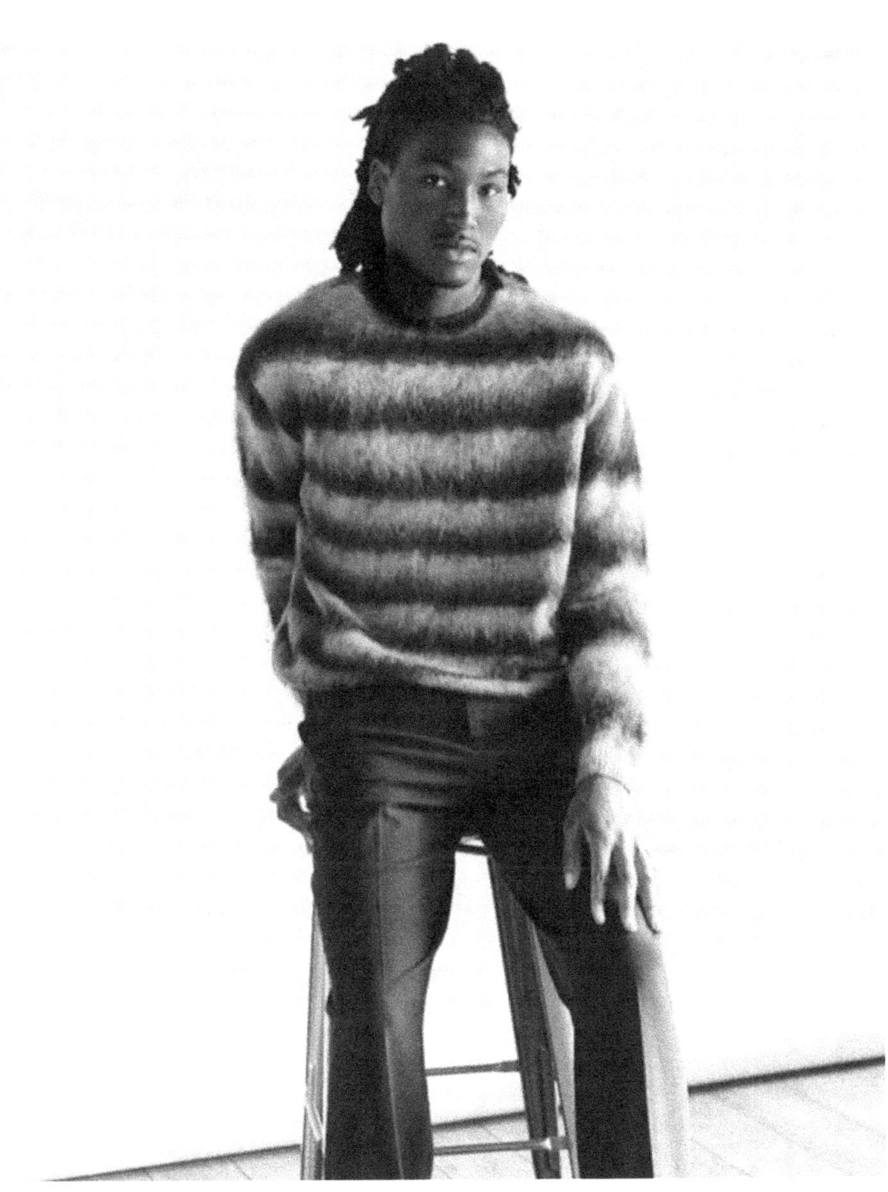